Slimming success. A comprehensive guide to a sustainable weight loss.

Vana Hendy.

DEDICATION

This book is dedicated to my family and friends and my Mentor Daniel who believed in me and supported me.Your love, encouragement, support has been my driving force throughout this journey, and I am immensely grateful for the role each of you played in bringing this book to life.

May these pages serve as a token of my appreciation and a small reflection of the impact you've had on my life. Thank you for being my Friends, family, mentors, inspiration. This book is as much yours as it is mine.

With heartfelt gratitude,

Vana Hendy.

CONTENTS

ACKNOWLEDGMENTS

I would like to express my heartfelt gratitude to the individuals who have played a significant role in the realization of this book. Their support, guidance, and encouragement have been invaluable.

First and foremost, I extend my deepest thanks to Almighty God for his love and mercy,I also want to thank my family and friends for their expertise, inspiration, encouragement.Your wisdom, insights, motivation significantly enriched this project.

I am also grateful to My Lecturers for their editorial assistance, feedback, support during challenging times.Your keen eye and thoughtful suggestions have greatly enhanced the quality of this work.

A special thanks to my mentor for his technical assistance and research support. Your dedication and expertise were instrumental in bringing this book to fruition.

Finally, a heartfelt thank you to my readers. Your interest in my work is the ultimate reward, and I am truly grateful for the opportunity to share this story with you.

Thank you all for being a part of this journey.

Sincerely,

Vana Hendy.

1 Understanding the Weight Loss Mindset

Introduction:
Achieving weight loss involves more than just following a diet plan or engaging in rigorous exercise. The mindset one adopts plays a crucial role in determining the success and sustainability of weight loss efforts. In this exploration, we delve into the various aspects of the weight loss mindset, emphasizing the importance of cultivating a positive and realistic approach for long-term success.

Shift from Short-Term Fixes to Lifestyle Changes:
Many individuals approach weight loss with a focus on quick fixes and immediate results. However, adopting a sustainable mindset

requires a shift from short-term fixes to embracing long-term lifestyle changes. This involves making healthier food choices, incorporating regular physical activity, and understanding that lasting results take time.

Set Realistic and Attainable Goals:
Unrealistic expectations can lead to frustration and disappointment. The weight loss mindset should involve setting realistic and attainable goals. Instead of fixating on a specific number on the scale, consider focusing on behavior-based goals such as incorporating more vegetables into meals, increasing daily steps, or practicing mindful eating.

Embrace a Positive Self-Image:
A healthy weight loss mindset involves fostering a positive self-image. Constant self-criticism and negative thoughts can undermine motivation and self-discipline. Acceptance of oneself at every stage of the journey, coupled with a belief in the ability to make positive changes, is essential for long-term success.

Learn from Setbacks:

Weight loss is a journey with inevitable ups and downs. Individuals with a resilient mindset view setbacks as learning opportunities rather than failures. Understanding the reasons behind setbacks, adjusting strategies accordingly, and moving forward with renewed determination contribute to a positive weight loss mindset.

Prioritize Mental and Emotional Well-being:

Weight loss is not solely about physical transformation; mental and emotional well-being are equally important.Stress, emotional eating, and negative emotions can all affect weight loss attempts.Adopting mindfulness practices, seeking support from friends or professionals, and addressing emotional triggers are crucial aspects of the weight loss mindset.

Build Sustainable Habits:

The weight loss mindset involves building sustainable habits that contribute to overall well-being. Instead of focusing on restrictive diets, individuals should cultivate habits that can be maintained in the long run. This includes enjoying a balanced diet, staying active, and getting adequate sleep.

Celebrate Non-Scale Victories:
Beyond the scale, numerous victories mark a successful weight loss journey. Celebrate improvements in energy levels, increased stamina, better sleep, and enhanced mood. Recognizing and appreciating these non-scale victories reinforce positive behavior and contribute to a healthy mindset.

Seek Professional Guidance:
A weight loss journey can be challenging, and seeking guidance from healthcare professionals, dietitians, or fitness experts can provide valuable support. These experts can offer personalized advice, address specific concerns, and help individuals navigate the complexities of weight loss in a healthy and sustainable way.

Conclusion:
Understanding the weight loss mindset is fundamental to achieving lasting success in one's journey towards a healthier lifestyle. By

prioritizing realistic goals, fostering positive self-image, learning from setbacks, and embracing a holistic approach to well-being, individuals can cultivate a mindset that not only leads to weight loss but also contributes to overall health and happiness. Remember, it's not just about losing weight; it's about gaining a healthier and more fulfilling life.

introduction

The science of weight loss is a complex and multifaceted field that involves understanding the interplay of various biological, psychological, and environmental factors. Successful weight loss is not just about following a fad diet or engaging in intense exercise for a short period; it requires a comprehensive approach that considers lifestyle, behavior, and individual differences. Here are key aspects of the science of weight loss:

Caloric Balance:

Weight loss fundamentally revolves around the concept of caloric balance—calories in versus calories out. To lose weight, you need to consume fewer calories than your body expends. This can be accomplished by combining calorie restriction with increased physical activity.

Metabolism:

Your body requires a certain amount of energy at rest, known as basal metabolic rate (BMR). Understanding and optimizing your metabolism is crucial for weight loss. Factors such as age, gender, muscle mass, and genetics influence metabolism. Muscle tissue burns more calories than fat, so building and maintaining muscle through strength training can positively impact metabolism.

Nutrition:

A balanced and nutrient-dense diet is essential for weight loss.Give priority to whole foods, including fruits, vegetables, whole grains, lean meats, and healthy fats. Portion control is also crucial. Avoiding excessive intake of processed foods, sugary beverages, and high-calorie snacks can help manage overall calorie intake.

Behavioral Psychology:

Understanding and modifying eating behaviors is a key aspect of successful weight loss. This includes addressing emotional eating, developing mindful eating habits, and building a healthy relationship with food. Behavioral changes may involve setting realistic goals, creating positive habits, and finding effective coping mechanisms for stress.

Physical Activity:

Exercise on a regular basis is crucial for both weight loss and general health. Both aerobic exercise (e.g., walking, running, cycling) and resistance training contribute to burning calories and improving metabolism. Additionally, physical activity has numerous health benefits beyond weight loss, including improved mood, increased energy, and reduced risk of chronic diseases.

Hormonal Factors:

Hormones are important for controlling metabolism and hunger.Factors such as insulin, ghrelin, leptin, and cortisol influence hunger, satiety, and fat storage. Balancing these hormones through lifestyle changes, including proper nutrition and exercise, can support weight loss efforts.

Sleep and Stress:

Inadequate sleep and chronic stress can negatively impact weight loss. Poor sleep can disrupt hormonal balance and increase cravings for unhealthy foods, while chronic stress can lead to emotional eating. Prioritizing quality sleep and adopting stress management strategies are integral to a comprehensive weight loss plan.

Individual Variability:

Each person is unique, and there is no one-size-fits-all approach to weight loss. Factors such as genetics, medical conditions, and personal preferences influence how individuals respond to different interventions. Tailoring weight loss strategies to individual needs and preferences increases the likelihood of long-term success.

In conclusion, achieving and maintaining weight loss involves a holistic approach that addresses multiple factors. Consulting with healthcare professionals, including registered dietitians and fitness experts, can provide personalized guidance and support on the journey to a healthier weight. It's essential to focus on sustainable lifestyle changes rather than quick fixes for long-term success.

Creating a personalized weight loss plan is a crucial step toward achieving your fitness goals. A one-size-fits-all approach may not be effective since individuals have unique body types, lifestyles, and preferences. Here's a comprehensive guide to help you create a personalized weight loss plan:

Set Realistic Goals:

Establish achievable short-term and long-term goals.

Make goals specific, measurable, and time-bound.

Consider factors like weight loss target, fitness level, and health improvements.

Assess Your Current Lifestyle:

Analyze your current eating habits, exercise routine, and sleep patterns.

Identify areas for improvement and potential obstacles.

Consult a Healthcare Professional:

Before making significant changes, consult with a healthcare provider or a registered dietitian.

Discuss any underlying health conditions or dietary restrictions.

Create a Balanced Diet:

Give special attention to nutrient-dense, entire foods including fruits, vegetables, lean meats, and whole grains.

Monitor portion sizes and practice mindful eating.

To stay hydrated, sip lots of water throughout the day.

Plan Meals and Snacks:

Plan meals ahead to avoid unhealthy food choices.

Include a balance of macronutrients (proteins, fats, and carbohydrates) in each meal.

Opoints for more frequent, smaller meals that sustain energy levels.

Incorporate Regular Exercise:

Choose exercises you enjoy to make it sustainable.

Combine cardiovascular activities, strength training, and flexibility exercises.

As your fitness level increases, gradually up the duration and intensity.

Stay Consistent:

Consistency is key to long-term success.

Create a routine that works with your lifestyle and schedule.

Track your progress and make adjustments as needed.

Get Adequate Sleep:

Lack of sleep can hinder weight loss efforts.

Aim for 7-9 hours of quality sleep each night.

Manage Stress:

Engage in stress-
relieving exercises such as yoga, meditation, o
r deep breathing.

Chronic stress can contribute to weight gain, so it's crucial to manage it effectively.

Monitor and Adjust:

Keep a food and exercise journal to track your

habits.

Review your objectives on a regular basis and modify your plan as necessary.

Celebrate Achievements:

Celebrate small victories to stay motivated.

Focus on the positive changes you've made rather than setbacks.

Seek Support:

To keep yourself accountable, tell friends and family about your goals

Consider joining a fitness group or seeking guidance from a professional.

Be Patient and Persistent:

Weight loss takes time, and results may vary.

Stay committed to your plan, and don't be discouraged by temporary setbacks.

Remember, it's essential to tailor your weight loss plan to your individual needs and preferences. Regularly reassess and make adjustments as needed to ensure continued progress and overall well-being.

A healthy weight can be attained and maintai ned largely through nutrition Here are some essential guidelines for weight loss through proper nutrition:

Caloric Deficit:

The basic principle of weight loss is to consum e fewer calories than your body uses.   Create a calorie deficit by either reducing your calorie intake or increasing your physical activity.

Balanced Macronutrients:

Make sure your consumption of the macronu

trients—fats, proteins, and carbohydrates—is balanced. Each has a role in the body, and a balanced approach supports overall health.

Pay attention to complex carbs found in lean proteins, whole grains, and healthy fats.

Portion Control:

Be mindful of portion sizes. Overeating, even healthy foods, can contribute to excess calorie intake.

High-Fiber Foods:

Eat a lot of foods high in fiber, such as whole grains, legumes, fruits, and vegetables. Fiber promotes satiety, helping you feel full for longer.

Lean Proteins:

Prioritize lean protein sources like chicken, fish, tofu, beans, and legumes. Protein helps maintain muscle mass, supports metabolism, and contributes to the feeling of fullness.

Healthy Fats:

Incorporate foods like avocados, almonds, se eds, and olive oil that are rich in healthful fats . These fats are essential for overall health and can help control appetite.

Hydration:

Drink plenty of water throughout the day. Sometimes, the body may signal thirst as hunger, leading to unnecessary calorie consumption.

Limit Added Sugars and Processed Foods:

Reduce the intake of sugary beverages, sweets, and processed foods. These items are often high in empty calories and provide little nutritional value.

Meal Timing:

Consider spreading your meals throughout the day to maintain energy levels and prevent excessive hunger that might lead to overeating.

Mindful Eating:

Observe the signals of hunger and fullness your body sends you, Avoid distractions like watching TV while eating to promote mindful eating.

Regular Exercise:

Combine a healthy diet with regular physical activity for optimal weight loss results. Exercise provides many health advantages in addition to burning calories.

Gradual Changes:

Aim for gradual, sustainable changes rather than drastic diets. This promotes long-term adherence and helps avoid the pitfalls of yo-yo dieting.

Consult a Professional:

If possible, consult with a registered dietitian or nutritionist. They can provide personalized guidance based on your individual needs, preferences, and health status.

Be Patient and Consistent:

Weight loss takes time. Be patient and stay consistent with your healthy eating habits and lifestyle changes.

Remember, individual nutritional needs vary, and what works for one person may not work for another. It's crucial to find an approach that fits your lifestyle and preferences while ensuring you meet your nutritional requirements. Before making significant changes to your diet, it's advisable to consult with a healthcare professional or nutrition expert, especially if you have underlying health conditions.

Effective exercise strategies are crucial for achieving fitness goals, improving overall health, and maintaining a sustainable workout routine. Here are some key principles to consider when developing an effective exercise plan:

Set Clear Goals:

Establish SMART goals, which stand for specifi c, measurable, achievable, relevant, and time -bound.
Consider both short-term and long-term objectives, such as weight loss, muscle gain, or improved cardiovascular health.
Choose Activities You Enjoy:

Option for exercises that you find enjoyable, as this increases the likelihood of sticking to your routine.
Experiment with different activities to find what suits your preferences and fits into your lifestyle.

Create a Balanced Routine:

Include a variety of cardiovascular, strength,and flexibility activities.
Balance different types of workouts to target various muscle groups and energy systems.

Gradual Progression:

Start with an appropriate intensity and gradually increase the difficulty to avoid overtraining and reduce the risk of injury.
Use the principle of progressive overload by consistently challenging your body to adapt to new levels of stress.

Consistency is Key:

Establish a regular exercise schedule and

make it a habit.

Consistency is more important than intensity; a moderate, regular workout routine is often more sustainable than sporadic intense sessions.

Include Rest and Recovery:

Allow time for your body to recover between intense workouts to prevent burnout and reduce the risk of injuries.

Adequate sleep, hydration, and proper nutrition play crucial roles in recovery.

Warm-up and Cool Down:

Warm up your muscles and joints vigorously b efore each session to get them ready for exer cise.

Include a cool-down phase with static stretching to improve flexibility and aid in muscle recovery.

Listen to Your Body:

Observe how your body reacts to activity.
If you experience pain (not to be confused

with the discomfort of a challenging workout), fatigue, or other signs of overtraining, adjust your routine accordingly.

Mix It Up:

Keep your workouts interesting by introducing variety.
Try new exercises, workout classes, or outdoor activities to prevent boredom and stimulate different muscle groups.

Stay Hydrated and Eat Well:

Proper hydration is essential for optimal performance and recovery.
Maintain a balanced diet with an emphasis on nutrients that support your fitness goals.

Seek Professional Guidance:

Consult with fitness professionals, such as personal trainers or physical therapists, to create a customized exercise plan based on your individual needs and limitations.

Track Your Progress:

Keep a record of your workouts, noting improvements in strength, endurance, or other relevant metrics.

Tracking progress can provide motivation and help you make informed adjustments to your exercise routine.

Remember that the most effective exercise plan is one that aligns with your personal goals, preferences, and lifestyle. It's essential to find a balance that promotes physical well-being while being sustainable in the long term.

6 OVERCOMING WEIGHT LOSS CHALLENGES

Overcoming weight loss challenges can be a demanding journey, both physically and mentally. However, with determination, realistic goals, and a sustainable approach, you can achieve and maintain a healthy weight.

Here are some strategies to help you overcome weight loss challenges:

Set Realistic Goals: Start by setting achievable and realistic goals. Aim for gradual weight loss, such as 1-2 pounds per week. Unrealistic expectations can lead to frustration and abandonment of your weight loss efforts.

Create a Balanced Diet: Adopt a balanced and nutritious diet that includes a variety of foods. Focus on whole grains, lean proteins, fruits, vegetables, and healthy fats. Avoid extreme diets or restrictive eating habits, as they are often unsustainable.

Portion Control: Be mindful of portion sizes. Use smaller plates and bowls to help control your portions and prevent overeating. Pay attention to hunger and fullness cues, and eat slowly to allow your body to recognize when it's satisfied.

Stay Hydrated: Drinking water can help control hunger and support overall health. Sometimes, our bodies can mistake thirst for hunger.
Make it a point to stay hydrated during the da y by drinking enough water.

Regular Physical Activity: Engage in regular physical activity that you enjoy. Find activities that fit into your lifestyle and gradually increase the intensity and duration. Walking, running, swimming, cycling, and eve n dancing may fall under this category.

Consistency is Key: Weight loss takes time, and consistency is crucial. Avoid the temptation to rely on fad diets or extreme measures. Focus on making sustainable lifestyle changes that you can maintain in the long run.

Manage Stress: Stress can contribute to overeating and unhealthy food choices. Find effective stress management techniques such as meditation, yoga, deep breathing, or hobbies that bring you joy.

Get Adequate Sleep: Lack of sleep can disrupt your body's hunger hormones and lead to weight
gain.For the purpose of supporting general he alth and weight management, aim for 7-
9 hours of good sleep each night.

Build a Support System: Share your weight loss goals with friends or family who can provide support and encouragement.Having a solid support netwo rk can keep you accountable and motivated

Celebrate Small Wins: Acknowledge and celebrate your achievements along the way, no matter how small. This positive reinforcement can keep you motivated and focused on your long-term goals.

Seek Professional Guidance: If needed, consider consulting with a healthcare professional, nutritionist, or fitness trainer. They can offer tailored counsel and recommendations according to your particular requirements and state of health.

Remember, weight loss is a journey, and it's essential to approach it with patience and a positive mindset. Focus on making sustainable lifestyle changes that promote overall health and well-being.

7 BUILDING HEALTHY HABITS

Building healthy habits is a fundamental and empowering process that contributes significantly to overall well-being. Whether you're striving for physical fitness, mental wellness, or a balanced lifestyle, cultivating positive habits can lead to lasting positive change. Here are some key insights into building and maintaining healthy habits:

Start Small:
Begin with manageable, attainable goals. Setting small, realistic targets helps you build momentum and confidence. As you achieve these initial milestones, you can gradually increase the complexity of your habits.

Consistency is Key:
Consistency is crucial when forming habits. Regular, repeated actions create neural pathways in the brain, making it easier for the behavior to become automatic. Aim for daily or regular practice to reinforce your commitment.

Define Clear Goals:
Clearly define your goals to give your habits purpose. Whether it's improving fitness, enhancing mental clarity, or adopting a healthier diet, having a clear objective provides direction and motivation.

Understand the Why:
Identify the underlying reasons for wanting to develop a particular habit. Understanding the "why" reinforces your commitment and helps you stay motivated during challenging times.

Build a Routine:
Integrate your new habits into an existing routine. Linking them to established activities makes it easier to remember and incorporate into your daily life.

Track Your Progress:

Keep a record of your achievements. Tracking progress not only helps you stay motivated but also allows for reflection and adjustment of your approach if needed.

Be Patient and Persistent:

Habits take time to develop. Be patient with yourself, and don't get discouraged by setbacks. Persistence is key to overcoming obstacles and maintaining positive behaviors.

Surround Yourself with Support:

Tell those you work with, family, or friends ab out your goals so they can support and hold y ou accountable.

Your chances of success might be greatly incr eased by surrounding yourself with helpful pe ople.

Focus on One Habit at a Time:

It can be daunting to try to change too much at once. Concentrate on establishing one habit before moving on to the next. This approach fosters sustainable, long-term change.

Celebrate Successes:
Celebrate and acknowledge your accomplishments, no matter how small. Rewarding yourself reinforces the positive associations with your new habits and boosts your motivation.

Adapt and Evolve:
Life is dynamic, and your habits may need to adapt accordingly. Be open to adjusting your approach based on changing circumstances or personal growth.

Prioritize Self-Care:
Building healthy habits goes hand in hand with self-care. Ensure you get enough sleep, maintain a balanced diet, and manage stress levels. A holistic approach to well-being enhances the likelihood of successful habit formation.

Remember, the journey of building healthy habits is unique to each individual. Be kind to yourself, stay committed, and enjoy the transformative process as you cultivate a healthier and more fulfilling lifestyle.

Staying motivated for the long haul can be challenging, especially when faced with obstacles, setbacks, or the monotony of pursuing a long-term goal. However, maintaining motivation over an extended period is crucial for achieving sustained success. Here are some tips to help you stay motivated for the long haul:

Define Clear Goals:
Clearly define your long-term goals. Break them down into smaller, manageable steps. This not only makes the journey more achievable but also provides a roadmap for your progress.

Create a Vision Board:
Visualize your goals by creating a vision board. Use images, quotes, and symbols that represent your aspirations. Place it somewhere visible to serve as a daily reminder of what you're working towards.

Celebrate Small Wins:
Acknowledge and celebrate small achievements along the way. Recognizing your progress, no matter how minor, helps to boost your confidence and keeps you motivated for the next steps.

Maintain a Positive Mindset:
Cultivate a positive mindset by focusing on the opportunities and possibilities rather than dwelling on challenges. Train your mind to see setbacks as learning experiences and opportunities for growth.

Break it Down:
Break your long-term goal into smaller, more manageable tasks.
This helps you focus on one stage at a time an d lessens the overall goal's overpowering qual ity.

Stay Flexible:
Be flexible in your approach. Sometimes the path to success may require adjustments. Embrace change and be willing to adapt your strategies as needed.

Surround Yourself with Support:
Build a support network of friends, family, or colleagues who encourage and believe in your abilities. Share your goals with them, and lean on them for support during challenging times.

Keep Learning:
Continuous learning can be a powerful motivator. Stay curious and seek new knowledge related to your goals. This not only enhances your skills but also keeps your enthusiasm alive.

Maintain a Healthy Lifestyle:
Physical well-being directly affects mental well-
being.Make sure you eat a balanced diet, exe rcise frequently, and get adequate sleep.A healthy body contributes to a healthy mind.

Reflect Regularly:

Take time to reflect on your journey. Evaluate your progress, reevaluate your goals if necessary, and appreciate the lessons learned along the way. Reflection helps you stay focused and aligned with your aspirations.

Visualize Success:

Spend time visualizing your success. Imagine achieving your long-term goals in vivid detail. This mental imagery can serve as a powerful motivator and reinforce your commitment.

Set Milestones:

Break down your long-term goal into smaller milestones. Celebrate each milestone as it brings you closer to your ultimate objective, providing a sense of accomplishment and motivation to keep going.

Remember that staying motivated for the long haul is a dynamic process that requires dedication, resilience, and a commitment to personal growth. By implementing these strategies, you can foster the resilience needed to overcome challenges and keep moving forward toward your long-term goals.

Sustaining weight loss for a lifetime involves adopting healthy habits, making lifestyle changes, and cultivating a positive mindset. While many people can successfully lose weight in the short term, maintaining that weight loss over the long term requires ongoing commitment and a holistic approach. Here are some key strategies to help you sustain weight loss for a lifetime:

Set Realistic Goals:
Establish achievable and realistic weight loss goals. Unrealistic goals can lead to frustration and discouragement.

Focus on Long-Term Lifestyle Changes:
Avoid quick fixes or extreme diets. Instead,

focus on making sustainable changes to your lifestyle, including dietary habits and physical activity.

Balanced Nutrition:

Emphasize a balanced diet with a variety of nutrient-dense

foods.Include entire grains, fruits, vegetables, lean meats, and healthy fats in your meals.

Portion Control:

Be mindful of portion sizes. Use smaller plates, listen to your body's hunger cues, and avoid overeating.

Regular Physical Activity:

Include regular exercise in your routine. To incorporate fitness into your lifestyle on a l ong-

term basis, engage in things you enjoy.Aim for at least 150 minutes of moderate-intensity exercise per week.

Build Healthy Habits:

Cultivate healthy habits such as mindful eating, staying hydrated, and getting adequate sleep.

These routines assist in maintaining a healthy weight and enhance general wellbeing.

Stay Hydrated:

Drink plenty of water throughout the day.

Sometimes, our bodies can mistake thirst for hunger.

 Monitor and Adjust:

Keep a close eye on your development and ad apt as necessary If you notice weight fluctuations, revisit your habits and make necessary changes.

Manage Stress:

Develop effective stress-management strategies, as stress can contribute to emotional eating and disrupt healthy habits.

 Social Support:

Surround yourself with supportive friends and family. Share your goals with them, and seek their encouragement. Joining a weight loss or fitness group can provide additional support.

 Celebrate Non-Scale Victories:

Acknowledge and celebrate achievements beyond the scale, such as improved energy levels, increased fitness, or better sleep.

 Mindful Eating:

Practice mindful eating by paying attention to your food, savoring each bite, and eating without distractions. This can help prevent overeating.

 Regular Health Check-Ups:

Schedule regular check-ups with your

healthcare provider to monitor your overall health and address any potential issues promptly.

Learn from Setbacks:
Understand that setbacks may happen. Instead of dwelling on them, learn from the experience and use it as an opportunity to adjust your approach.

Cultivate a Positive Mindset:
Adopt a positive and realistic mindset. Understand that weight loss is a journey with ups and downs, and maintaining a healthy weight is a lifelong commitment.

Conclusion:
Sustaining weight loss for a lifetime is about adopting a balanced and sustainable approach to nutrition, exercise, and overall well-being. It involves making long-term lifestyle changes, building healthy habits, and developing a positive mindset. By incorporating these strategies into your daily life, you increase your chances of not only losing weight but also maintaining it for the long haul.

Develop strategies for maintaining your weight loss achievements and transitioning into a sustainable, long-term healthy lifestyle.

Bonus Recipes and Meal Plans

Enjoy a selection of delicious and nutritious recipes, along with sample meal plans to make healthy eating an enjoyable and sustainable part of your life.

Empower yourself with the knowledge and tools needed to achieve lasting weight loss success. "Slimming Success" is your roadmap to a healthier, happier, and more confident you. Start your journey today.

ABOUT THE AUTHOR

Vana Hendy is a seasoned wordsmith with a passion for storytelling that has captivated readers around the world. Born and raised in Nigeria, Vana Hendy discovered the magic of words at an early age, weaving tales that transported readers to fantastical realms and stirred their imaginations.

With a degree in Marketing from Coal City University , Vana Hendy combines a strong academic foundation with a natural flair for creative expression. This unique blend of knowledge and creativity is evident in her ability to craft narratives that are both intellectually stimulating and emotionally resonant.

Vana Hendy has a diverse literary palette, having penned works spanning various genres, from gripping mystery novels to heartwarming romance stories. she believes in the transformative power of storytelling, using words to inspire, entertain, and provoke thought.